**Cibangu Katamba**

**Attending antenatal care at the hospital versus clinic**

AF153287

Cibangu Katamba

# Attending antenatal care at the hospital versus clinic

## Averting the risk of late repeat caesarean section

**LAP LAMBERT Academic Publishing**

**Impressum / Imprint**

Bibliografische Information der Deutschen Nationalbibliothek: Die Deutsche Nationalbibliothek verzeichnet diese Publikation in der Deutschen Nationalbibliografie; detaillierte bibliografische Daten sind im Internet über http://dnb.d-nb.de abrufbar.
Alle in diesem Buch genannten Marken und Produktnamen unterliegen warenzeichen-, marken- oder patentrechtlichem Schutz bzw. sind Warenzeichen oder eingetragene Warenzeichen der jeweiligen Inhaber. Die Wiedergabe von Marken, Produktnamen, Gebrauchsnamen, Handelsnamen, Warenbezeichnungen u.s.w. in diesem Werk berechtigt auch ohne besondere Kennzeichnung nicht zu der Annahme, dass solche Namen im Sinne der Warenzeichen- und Markenschutzgesetzgebung als frei zu betrachten wären und daher von jedermann benutzt werden dürften.

Bibliographic information published by the Deutsche Nationalbibliothek: The Deutsche Nationalbibliothek lists this publication in the Deutsche Nationalbibliografie; detailed bibliographic data are available in the Internet at http://dnb.d-nb.de.
Any brand names and product names mentioned in this book are subject to trademark, brand or patent protection and are trademarks or registered trademarks of their respective holders. The use of brand names, product names, common names, trade names, product descriptions etc. even without a particular marking in this work is in no way to be construed to mean that such names may be regarded as unrestricted in respect of trademark and brand protection legislation and could thus be used by anyone.

Coverbild / Cover image: www.ingimage.com

Verlag / Publisher:
LAP LAMBERT Academic Publishing
ist ein Imprint der / is a trademark of
OmniScriptum GmbH & Co. KG
Heinrich-Böcking-Str. 6-8, 66121 Saarbrücken, Deutschland / Germany
Email: info@lap-publishing.com

Herstellung: siehe letzte Seite /
Printed at: see last page
**ISBN: 978-3-659-71149-7**

Zugl. / Approved by: United Kingdom, Manchester Metropolitan University, Dissertation, April 2014

# TABLE OF CONTENT

SUMMARY

The global maternal deaths were approximately 287 000 in 2010 according to the World Health organization fact sheet (May 2012) on maternal mortality. Most of these maternal mortalities occurred in developing settings.

In Zambia, many maternal deaths could be prevented; home deliveries are high and account for 53% against 47% of deliveries at health facility (assisted by skilled personnel). Young child mortality though declining is still a burden. According to the United Nations Children's Fund (UNICEF) report, the mortality rates (neonate, infant and under five) are still high and unacceptable.

The 2007 Zambian demographic health survey revealed that about 94% of mothers received antenatal care (ANC) from skilled health workers. About 99% of women living in urban areas received ANC (nearly universal ANC) from skilled providers as opposed to 91% of women in rural areas. From the same source, caesarean section deliveries were rated at 3 %.

Since most hospitals in Zambia offer Emergency Obstetric and neonatal Care (EmOC) as opposed to Urban health centres (clinics); the aim of this study is to establish if mothers who have had a previous caesarean section have a chance of improving their health and that of their new born infants by attending ANC at the hospital compared with those who attend at the clinic. The study will review medical records of consecutive delivery for women with previous caesarean section who were followed up antenatally at Ndola Central Hospital (NCH) and of those referred to NCH from the surrounding clinics between January 2011 and December 2012.

Data availability in developing settings is scarce: previous rates of caesarean section and how much this varies by year and geographic areas are limited. Previous studies comparing ANC in previous caesarean mothers between hospital and clinic are lacking in developed countries. Emergency caesareans are often performed too late to cut down perinatal mortalities in developing settings.

The present study proposes to compare the rates of late emergency repeat caesarean section between attending ANC at the hospital and at the clinic for women who have had a previous caesarean delivery. The primary objective of this study is to establish if attending ANC at the hospital protects mothers with previous caesarean section from late access to emergency repeat caesarean section. The study will also seek to establish if late access to emergency repeat caesarean section is associated with increased rate of stillbirths.

A retrospective cohort study methodology will be used. A total number of 544 exposed subjects (about 318 records) and 544 unexposed subjects (about 318 records) for the duration of two years (from 2011 to 2012) will be reviewed. The uncorrected Chi-squared statistic will be used to evaluate the null hypothesis. Data will be analysed using Epi Info version 7.

## BACKGROUND

There were about 287,000 maternal deaths in 2010 globally[1]. For every maternal death, more women are affected by disabilities, injuries and infections[1]. Developing countries account for about 99% of all maternal deaths[1]. The risk of dying during childbirth is highest in sub-Saharan Africa and southern Asia (most women give birth without skilled care) [2].

Many maternal deaths could be prevented. In my settings (Zambia), 47% of deliveries only are assisted by skilled health personnel at health settings [2]. The deliveries at home are still high and account for 53% of the total; there are inequalities in the risk of maternal death; in rural settings communities have limited access to health care services[2]. Approximately 99% of the population are within 5 kilometres of health care facilities in urban settings, compared to only 50% in rural settings[2] Socio-culturally, health care seeking behaviours for families are such that pregnancy is not given special care in Zambia. All these factors contribute to high maternal mortality. Haemorrhage, sepsis, obstructed labour, hypertensive disorders; abortion, malaria and HIV are the leading causes of maternal death in Zambia[3]. According to the United Nations Children's Fund (UNICEF) report[4], young child mortality in Zambia, though declining, is still a burden. The mortality rates (neonate, infant and under five) are still high and unacceptable[4]. The Zambian ministry of health, UNICEF and World Health Organization (WHO) analysis on child health situation suggest that the key child survival interventions in Zambia are inadequate to achieve the required reduction of child mortality[5].

According to the 2007 Zambian demographic health survey[6], about 94% of mothers received antenatal care (ANC) from skilled health workers. About 99% of women living in urban areas received ANC (nearly universal ANC) from skilled providers as opposed to 91% of women in rural areas[6]. From the same source, caesarean section deliveries were rated at 3 %. Caesarean deliveries were more frequent among highly educated women, women living in urban settings, and women at first delivery[6]. In a cross-sectional study conducted by Paulo Souza Joao and colleagues[7], having had a previous caesarean section among other high risk factors was associated with severe maternal morbidity, very low and low birth weight, early neonatal morbidity and mortality, stillbirth, prolonged maternal stay in the hospital after delivery and repeat caesarean section.

There are about 1,956 healthcare facilities in Zambia[8]. The government runs about 85% of these facilities, the private sector and missions (religious affiliated) run 9% and 6% respectively[9]. There are five levels of public health facilities in the Zambian healthcare system[8]: a) third level hospitals (specialist or tertiary/ central hospitals), highest referral hospitals in the nation; b) second level hospitals (provincial or general hospitals), acting as referrals for first level hospitals; c) first level hospitals (or district hospitals), acting as referrals for health centres; d) health centres (are of two types at the community level), including urban health centres also called **clinics** and rural health centres; and e) health posts (lowest level of healthcare), offering only basic first aid care. Almost all hospitals offer emergency obstetric care (EmOC) in Zambia while most clinics (urban health centres) do not[8].

This study will seek to establish if mothers who have had a previous caesarean section have a chance of improving their health and that of their new born infants by attending ANC at the hospital compared with those who attend at the clinic. It will be a retrospective cohort study. Medical records of consecutive delivery for women with previous caesarean section who were followed up antenatally at Ndola Central Hospital (NCH) and of those referred to NCH from the surrounding clinics (between January 2011 and December 2012) will be reviewed.

## LITERATURE REVIEW

### Research question:

Can attending antenatal care at the hospital for mothers with previous caesarean delivery improve maternal and perinatal survival as compared to attending ANC at the clinic?

Construction of a searchable question using PICO:

| P | Mothers with previous caesarean delivery in Ndola district |
|---|---|
| I | Attending ANC at the hospital |
| C | Attending ANC at the clinic |
| O | Improved maternal and perinatal health: |
| |    1.  Reduced maternal morbidity and mortality |
| |    2.  Reduced perinatal morbidity and mortality |
| |    3.  Reduced risk of late emergency repeat caesarean section |

Table 1: PICO question

### Search strategy:

To review current knowledge of the above searchable question, quantitative and qualitative studies were reviewed in the already published literature. The search was conducted in Science Direct, PubMed and Google Scholar databases to identify suitable and accessible peer-reviewed English articles published between January 1995 and September 2013. The reference list and citations of the identified articles were also consulted to increase the reviewed results. Published literature of perinatology seminars was also included.

The selected articles for further review contained at least one of the following search terms: antenatal care after caesarean delivery OR previous caesarean delivery, hospital OR clinic, improving maternal and perinatal health, previous caesarean section OR repeat caesarean section, and Zambia. The review was further refined for Google Scholar database to reach a more manageable (but, as representative and exhaustive as possible) number of articles; including only articles focused on the interventions (PICO). The included Mesh terms were: "prenatal care" OR "antenatal care" AND "after" OR "previous" AND "caesarean section" OR "caesarean delivery" AND "improving" AND "mothers" OR "women" AND "maternal" AND "perinatal" AND " repeat" AND "caesarean section".

 A total number of 31 articles were selected after screening for duplication and relevance. Almost all the studies reviewed were conducted in developing countries, the majority being from Africa. Zambia has a high number of reviewed records (three) per single country. Most studies were recently published (between 2007 and 2013).

## Literature research flow chart:

The following literature review flow chart was constructed following the PRISMA 2009 flow diagram model.[10]

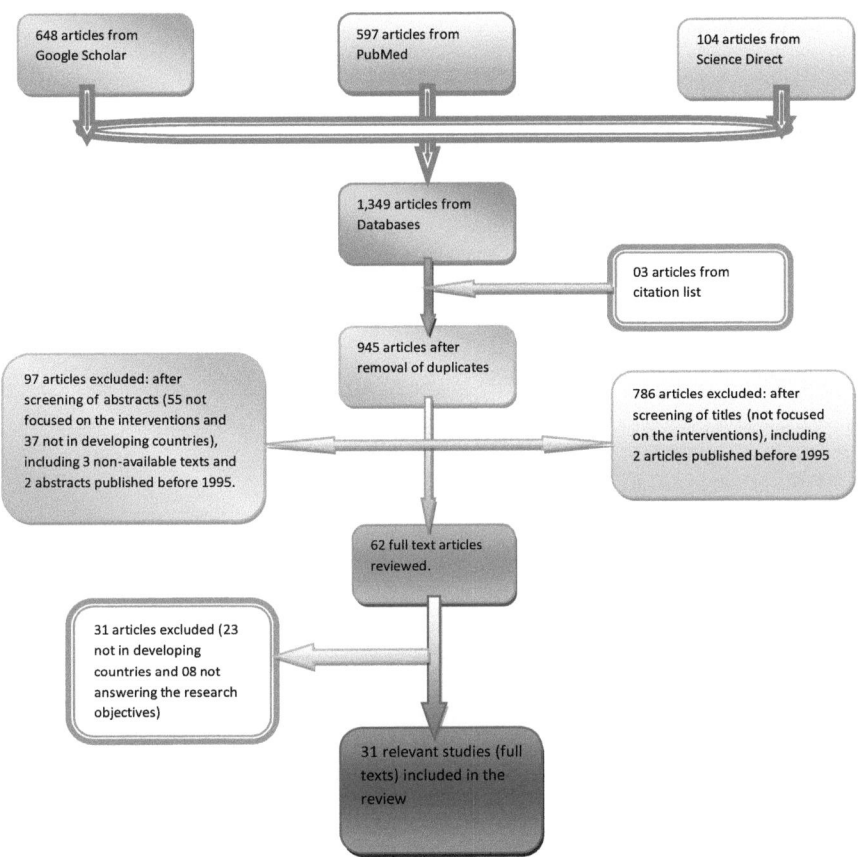

Figure 1: literature review flow diagram

## Summary of reviewed records by type:

| Type of study | Number of records |
|---|---|
| Systematic reviews and meta-analysis | 2 |
| Cluster randomised controlled trials | 1 |
| Cohort studies | 2 |
| Prospective descriptive studies | 1 |
| Case-control studies | 2 |
| Cross sectional and population based studies | 13 |
| Seminars in perinatology | 2 |
| Review of hospital records | 1 |
| Case scenario | 1 |
| Literature reviews | 6 |

Table 2: summary of reviewed articles by type

## Synthesis of reviewed articles by conclusions:

Having had a previous caesarean delivery predisposes pregnant women to perinatal and maternal complications risks in spite of her choice of mode of delivery (elective trial of labour or repeat caesarean section) [11]. Antenatal care, when used correctly to detect complications, educate pregnant women to discern danger signs in pregnancy, advise and motivate pregnant women (including their families) on the suitable time and place to seek referral care (within and to emergency obstetric and neonatal care: EmONC facilities) can contribute effectively to maternal and perinatal death reduction.[12-16]

Counselling pregnant women with previous caesarean section during antenatal care should be individualized to their circumstances and should discuss or provide the followings[11,17]:

- Complete, informed, detailed consent on risks and benefits of each mode of delivery;
- The risk of uterine rupture;
- The likelihood of successful vaginal birth after caesarean (VBAC);
- Future maternity plans;
- Possible risk of repeat caesarean delivery

Most clinics in Zambia do not offer caesarean section services. The majority of hospitals offer trial of scar (trial of labour in previous caesarean section) and elective caesarean section (including emergency caesarean section) services depending on each patient' clinical presentation.

The table below compares and contrasts the possibility of trial of labour in previous caesarean delivery and elective repeat caesarean delivery[11,17-23]:

| Trial of labour in previous caesarean delivery | Elective repeat caesarean delivery |
|---|---|
| ▪ Increased but less common risk of perinatal death and birth asphyxia | ▪ Less serious but frequent risk of neonatal risks: respiratory morbidity, cost and length of stay in the hospital |
| ▪ Additional attributable risk of about 0.25% of serious harmful perinatal outcomes at term for planned VBAC (NICHD study)[17] | ▪ This additional attributable risk of perinatal morbidity and mortality is reduced significantly or even eliminated for elective repeat caesarean section |
| ▪ Risk of uterine rupture<br>▪ Most trial of labour will be successful<br>▪ Failed VBAC increases the risk of birth injury, sepsis, and need for resuscitation. Failed VBAC can resolve in intra-partum | |

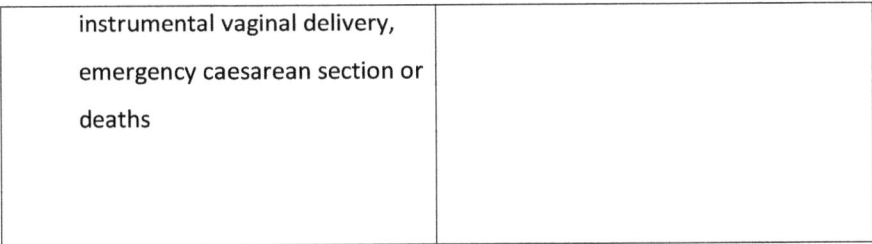

| instrumental vaginal delivery, emergency caesarean section or deaths | |
|---|---|
| | |

Table 4: trial of labour in previous caesarean Vs elective caesarean delivery

**Risks associated with late emergency repeat caesarean section:**

There is limited use of caesarean delivery in Africa[24]. When performed; emergency caesareans are in most cases too late to cut down perinatal mortalities[24].

Risk factors associated with perinatal mortality such as multiple pregnancy, previous caesarean section and breech presentation have been described[25]. Most perinatal deaths are stillbirths[20]. Improving the quality and utilisation of antenatal care combined with quality intra-partum care can reduce significantly perinatal mortality[26].

In a study conducted in Afghanistan[13], it was established that referral care provided in time to emergency obstetric and neonatal care facilities reduces the number of late emergency caesarean section. Focused efforts on improved quality of care are also needed to be made available and to reduce mortality.

## Importance of antenatal care:

The reviewed literature suggests that well conducted antenatal care reduces maternal mortality and morbidity through direct detection and management of illness during pregnancy or indirect detection of high risk pregnancy and assuring that women deliver at well equipped and appropriate health facility[27]. Research conducted in Kenya[28] and Bangladesh[29] revealed a positive association between antenatal care attendance with increased delivery at health facility and improved perinatal outcomes. On the other hand, inadequate antenatal care was found to be associated with increased obstetric complications[30].

## Barriers to utilization of antenatal care:

Below are listed identified obstacles to utilization of antenatal care in the reviewed literature[31-40]:

- Limited understanding of the importance of antenatal care
- Lack of awareness on standards of antenatal care
- Lack of information on quality of care to expect
- Lack of family support and community involvement, seeking permission
- Financial and transport challenges (long distance to health facility)
- Low education level
- High parity women (having delivered several times)
- Young mothers (aged 20 to 25 years)
- Cultural beliefs such as witchcraft
- Unplanned pregnancies

- Low socioeconomic status, poverty

- Shortages of care providers and staff insufficiency

- Negative attitude of health care providers toward the clients

- Lack of equipments at health facilities

- Non-availability of antenatal care services at primary health care level

In a study conducted in Niger by Prual and colleagues[31], it was established that quality antenatal care for risk factors screening was poor; midwives did not screen systematically for risk factors, including age, height, blood pressure, sugar levels in urine, swelling (of feet, hands or face), parity, bleeding per vagina, previous caesarean section, stillbirths and miscarriages in previous pregnancies. This situation is common in most developing settings.

## GAPS IN EXISTING LITERATURE

Programs investing in health infrastructure, health personnel and research can save lives. Health education aiming at promoting focused antenatal care services uptake need to be intensified to achieve improved perinatal and maternal health. Standardization and provision of information about antenatal care to women and their families requires attention by policy makers and health care providers. Education of both women and their husbands on the importance of antenatal care needs to be strengthened to achieve improved maternal and child health. Financial support is also important to achieve improved antenatal care services utilization[17]. There is need to improve socioeconomic status and literacy for women[17].

Risk factors associated with perinatal mortality including multiple pregnancy, previous caesarean section and breech presentation have been described[25]. Previous caesarean delivery is associated with maternal and perinatal complications regardless of choice of mode of delivery[26]. Data availability in developing countries is scarce: previous rates of caesarean section and how much this varies by year and geographic areas are limited. There is also a gap in the existing Zambian national data on antenatal care coverage[41], calling for focused quality antenatal care. Previous studies comparing antenatal care in previous caesarean between hospital and clinic are lacking in developing countries. This is worthwhile for further investigations. Further, randomized controlled trials among pregnant women undergoing a trial of labour after caesarean and longitudinal cohort studies among pregnant women with previous caesarean are needed to appraise adverse outcomes with focused attention on both infant and the mother. Interventions aiming at improving perinatal and maternal survival in previous caesarean section such as emergency obstetric and neonatal care (offered in hospital settings in Zambia) and focused quality antenatal care are encouraged (project proposal).


## RESEARCH TOPIC

The key research question is: can attending ANC at the hospital for mothers with previous caesarean section improve maternal and perinatal health as compared to attending ANC at the clinic in Ndola urban district of Zambia?

The research hypotheses are formulated as follows. The null hypothesis (Ho) = there is no statistically significant difference in rates of late emergency repeat caesarean section(1) and stillbirths(2) between attending ANC at the hospital(5% and 1% respectively) and attending ANC at the clinic(60% and 5% respectively) for mothers with previous caesarean delivery. The alternative hypothesis (H1) = there is statistically significant improved access to timely emergency repeat caesarean section (fewer late emergency repeat caesarean section) and fewer stillbirths for mothers with previous caesarean delivery who attend ANC at the hospital as compared to those who attend ANC at the clinic.

Study objectives: To ascertain if mothers who have had a previous caesarean section have a chance of improving their health and that of their new born infants by attending ANC at the hospital compared with those who attend at the clinic. The research will determine the extent to which maternal and child health are improved by attending ANC at the hospital for mothers with previous caesarean delivery. This will help to formulate recommendations to enable subsequent intervention to address the problem in health services delivery. Primarily, the study will seek to establish if attending ANC at the hospital protects mothers with previous caesarean delivery from late access to emergency repeat caesarean section. Secondly, the study will seek to establish if late access to emergency repeat caesarean section increases significantly the rates of stillbirths.

## STUDY DESIGN

This research will be a retrospective cohort study. Medical records of consecutive delivery for women with previous caesarean section who were followed up antenatally at Ndola Central Hospital (NCH) and of those referred to NCH from the surrounding clinics (between January 2011 and December 2012) will be reviewed. The groups of participants to be compared will be identified at the start of the study and defined as follows. Group 1: ANC at the clinic (these mothers were not availed of timely emergency obstetric and neonatal care = exposed); Group 2: ANC at the hospital (these mothers were availed of timely emergency obstetric and neonatal care = unexposed). Then, the researcher will look back (after follow up) to determine whether the subjects subsequently developed the outcomes of interest. This study will seek to establish if mothers who have had a previous caesarean section have a chance of improving their health and that of their new born infants by attending ANC at the hospital compared with those who attend at the clinic.

Choice of methodology: the retrospective cohort study design would be more appropriate in this case. It will identify and define groups to be compared at the start of the study as being from the hospital or from the clinic (exposure) and then look at the outcomes already observed (increased maternal and perinatal morbidity and mortality in the group of mothers attending ANC at the clinic = outcomes); and seek to address the problem (of maternal and perinatal ill health) in health services. This study is limited to those who delivered at the hospital in the group of those who attended antenatal care at the clinic (not including those who attended antenatal care and delivered at the clinic). In case of confounders, multivariate analysis and logistic regression will be used.

Justification: the rationale for choosing this study design lies in that cost can be reduced and time can be saved by using a historical cohort study. A longitudinal prospective cohort study may be a suitable alternative, but expensive and long term study. Randomised controlled trial may be unethical (depriving a group of women from emergency obstetric care).

Outcomes:

This research will assess whether there is significant improved health outcomes in the group of mothers with previous caesarean delivery who attended antenatal care at the hospital in Ndola urban district of Zambia. The expected maternal outcomes are: reduced morbidity (such as postpartum haemorrhage, uterine rupture, fistulas, sepsis, late emergency repeat caesarean section, and other injuries) and reduced mortality. The perinatal outcomes such as reduction in: birth asphyxia, fresh stillbirth, macerated stillbirth, and early neonatal death are expected. For this research, the outcomes of interest are timely emergency repeat caesarean section and fewer stillbirths in the group of unexposed mothers. It is known that elective caesarean sections are offered in specific patients for those attending ANC at the hospital. It is then expected to have timely emergency repeat caesarean section in this group; also, timely management of complications such as post partum haemorrhage and uterine rupture to avert deaths.


## TARGET POPULATION

Zambia is located in the south of sub-Saharan Africa and covers about 752,612 $km^2$. It is a landlocked country surrounded by 8 neighbouring countries: Tanzania and DR Congo in the north; Mozambique and Malawi in the east; Namibia, Zimbabwe and Botswana in the south; and Angola in the west. There is rapid growth of the Zambian population from about 3 million (in 1964) to 13.2 million people in 2010[11]. This burdens the national economy, especially the country's capacity to answer the health needs of a rapidly growing population. Zambia has 10 provinces; including: Central, Copperbelt, Eastern, Luapula, Lusaka, Muchinga, Northern, North-western, Southern, and Western provinces. Ndola is the provincial headquarters of the Copperbelt province. It is the third largest city of Zambia. Ndola district is mostly urban and peri-urban and covers about 110,300 hectares. As per the 2000 Zambia' national census, Ndola district had a population of 374,757. Ndola district has two third level hospitals: Arthur Davison Hospital (a children's hospital) and Ndola central hospital. The district has one first level hospital (Hill Top hospital, a private hospital), 43 urban health centres or clinics, and one rural health centre. Ndola central hospital serves as a referral in the district, province and surrounding provinces. Ndola central hospital is now serving a population of 503,649 in Ndola district.[42] it has a capacity of 851 beds and 97 cots.

The target population is women of reproductive age who have had a previous caesarean delivery and residing in Ndola district. The study population will be all mothers who have had a previous caesarean section and were followed up antenatally for consecutive delivery at Ndola central hospital or any clinic in Ndola district.

Inclusion criteria (the choice of exposed and unexposed subjects will be done as follows). Group 1 (exposed to lack of timely emergency obstetric and neonatal care): will comprise all women with one or more previous caesarean section(s) _being referred to NCH from the local clinic for consecutive delivery (ANC at the clinic); Group 2 (availed of timely emergency obstetric and neonatal care): will comprise all women with one or more previous caesarean section(s) _self referred from home to Ndola central hospital for consecutive delivery (ANC at the hospital).

It may be difficult to find all subjects whose records are going to be examined to obtain informed consent. The researcher has then the obligation to provide to the Ndola central hospital research ethical committee assurances that confidentiality will be maintained.

## SAMPLE SIZE AND SAMPLING PROCESS

This study will seek to establish if mothers who have had a previous caesarean section have a chance of improving their health and that of their new born infants by attending ANC at the hospital compared with those at the clinic. Health records of consecutive delivery for women with previous caesarean section who were followed up antenatally at Ndola Central Hospital and of those referred to NCH from the surrounding clinics will be reviewed.

According to the 2007 Zambian Demographic Health Survey, about 94% of mothers received ANC from skilled workers. About 99% of women living in urban areas received nearly universal ANC from skilled providers. From the same source, caesarean deliveries were rated at 3 percent. The proportions of caesarean section were higher in Copperbelt province (7 percent) and Lusaka province (6 percent) than in other provinces (1% to 3%).

Assuming that there will be an increase of caesarean section rate in Ndola of 5% (from 7% to 12%) by January 2010, the rate of mothers with previous caesarean delivery will be greater than 12% by January 2011 ( $\geq$ 13%). Most hospitals offer Emergency Obstetric and Neonatal Care (EmONC) services as opposed to clinics in Zambia. The crude birth rate in Zambia was 45, 56 per 1,000 people in 2010 according to World Bank[43]. This translates to (45, 56 births X 503,649 population in Ndola district)/1,000 people = 22,946 births in Ndola district in 2010. According to the 2007 Zambian Demographic Health survey, 52% of births occur at home and 48% at a health facility. This translates in 11,932 births at home and 11,014 births at health facility. Thirteen percent caesarean section rate of 11,014 births = 1,432 births per year and 2,864 births per two years (study duration).

Assumptions:

- About half the total caesarean section deliveries are referrals: there will be 1,432 caesarean section from the clinics (exposed) and 1,432 caesarean section from NCH (unexposed)
- About two-firth of the total caesarean deliveries are repeated caesarean deliveries: there will be 573 repeat caesarean section from the clinics (exposed) and 573 repeat caesarean section from NCH (unexposed)
- Ndola central hospital (unexposed): about 10% of all repeat caesarean section are elective/planned = 57 repeat caesarean deliveries, and about 90% of all repeat caesarean section are emergency = 516 deliveries; planned repeat caesarean section may turn into emergency repeat caesarean section if labour starts before the planned date of delivery, this transforms in about 95% emergency repeat caesarean section.
- Clinics (exposed): about 95% of repeat caesarean section are emergency = 544 emergency repeat caesarean section from the clinics.

Expected outcomes:

- Clinics: 544 emergency repeat caesarean sections (60% late and 40% timely); and about 5% or more stillbirths out of the total repeat emergency caesarean section.
- Hospitals: 544 emergency repeat caesarean section (5% late and 95% timely); and about less than 1% stillbirths out of the total repeat emergency caesarean section

The calculated sample size using Fleis' formulas for unmatched cohort studies[44]: n = 13 (for outcome 1: late emergency repeat caesarean section) and n = 318 (for outcome2: stillbirths). This translates as follows. We are planning a retrospective cohort study with a ratio of 1 unexposed to 1 exposed. According to our expected outcomes, the rates of late emergency repeat caesarean section and stillbirths will be: 5% and 1% respectively among unexposed subjects; 60% and 5% respectively among exposed subjects. Therefore, we will need to study at least 13 records for outcome (1)/ 318 records for outcome (2) of exposed subjects and similarly for unexposed subjects. This will enable us to reject the null hypothesis that the rates of late emergency repeat caesarean section and stillbirths for women attending ANC at the clinics and those at the hospital are equal with probability (power) 0.8. The type I error probability associated with this test of the null hypothesis is 0.05. We will use an uncorrected Chi-squared statistic to evaluate this null hypothesis.

All the clinics will be reviewed. Since our "exposed" women come from different clinics, we may have an issue with cluster sampling. Therefore, the researcher may need to estimate the design effect first in a pilot study to calculate the sample size required.

## STUDY METHODS AND DATA COLLECTION

Data collection will comprise: information on age, parity, marital status, file number, education level, socio-economic level, ANC site, number of previous caesarean deliveries, inter-pregnancy intervals, pregnancy outcome (spontaneous vaginal delivery, instrumental vaginal delivery, planned repeat caesarean section, emergency repeat caesarean section), causes of repeat caesarean section, duration of labour (time when labour started, time when partograph was opened, time when repeat caesarean section was indicated, time when repeat caesarean section was performed), maternal outcomes (postpartum haemorrhage, uterine rupture, fistulas, fever/sepsis, other injuries, death), and perinatal outcomes (fresh stillbirth, macerated stillbirth, birth asphyxia/APGAR score, early neonatal death). This information will be collected by professional health workers using Excel sheet tool. As the above data is found on medical records safely kept by the hospital as well as all clinics, the researcher will be able to collect it. The records are securely kept in the hospital obstetric registry and various clinic registries. Data are collected in a standardised manner (information is collected consistently on well designed medical forms on patient' identity, motif of consultation or referral, history of the present complaint, past medical history, obstetrics and gynaecology history, social history, past surgical and family history, physical examination, management, outcomes of labour,etc.). This information will then be crosschecked with data from relevant registers such as labour ward register and theatre register for its validation. For women referred to NCH from various clinics, data is also verified at the primary source.


**Statistical analysis:**

The data will then be analysed after ensuring that potential confounders (such as: age, level of education, socioeconomic status, marital status) are controlled. All information will be analysed using Epi Info version 7. Both descriptive and comparative analysis will be done. Comparative analysis will include the uncorrected Chi-Square tests (with 80% power, 95% confidence intervals, and odds ratio) to evaluate the null hypothesis that rates of late emergency repeat caesarean section and stillbirths (5% and 1% respectively in the unexposed group; 60% and 5% respectively in the exposed group) are equal in both groups. If the researcher find that confounding has occurred, there will be need to apply multivariable logistic regression analysis to adjust for possible confounders.

## TIMEFRAME

The table below summarises the key research activities.

| MONTHS / ACTIVITIES | 1 | 2 | 3 | 4 | 5 | 6 | 7 | 8 |
|---|---|---|---|---|---|---|---|---|
| Finalize research proposal and submit for clearance | X | | | | | | | |
| Obtain ethical clearance | | X | | | | | | |
| Design data collection tools | | X | | | | | | |
| Secure funds for project | X | X | | | | | | |
| Identification and training of data collectors (professional health workers) | | | X | | | | | |

| | | | X | X | X | | | |
|---|---|---|---|---|---|---|---|---|
| Data collection | | | X | X | X | | | |
| Cross-checking of data and primary verification (data validation) | | | | X | X | | | |
| Data entry, cleaning and statistical analysis | | | X | X | X | X | | |
| Data analysis | | | | | | X | X | |
| Report writing and dissemination of preliminary findings | | | | | | | X | |
| Final report submission | | | | | | | | X |

Table 5: research activities timeframe

About 900 obstetric records can be accessed weekly. Out of these records, 117 deliveries (by caesarean section) records may be screened for eligibility every week. Approximately 47 repeat caesarean section obstetric records will be screened for eligibility weekly. This translates to a total of 12 weeks (3 months) to complete the collection of all required data.

## ETHICAL CONSIDERATIONS

Permission to conduct this study will be sought and obtained from the Zambian Ministry of Health through the NCH research ethical committee and the provincial medical officer (who is also responsible for all the clinics in the province). Since it may be impractical to locate subjects whose records are going to be examined to obtain informed consent, the researcher has an obligation to provide to the ethical review committee assurances that confidentiality will be maintained.

Data will be collected from patients' records (by trained professional health workers) and cross-checked with information kept in relevant registers of deliveries in labour ward and operating theatre. To sensibly minimize potential biases such as information bias, verification of the information at the primary source (clinics for women referred to NCH) will also be done. The researcher will ensure that all data source documents are fully completed with all of the relevant information before being reported. All data collectors will be trained on how to use the data collection tool in view of accurate recording of information.

All information will be kept confidential and the identities of participants (exposed and unexposed) will not be disclosed in the report. The results of the research will be shared with participating institutions in order to maximize its benefits.

Women who visit the hospital are those living near the hospital or those who work/whose family members work at NCH. Women residing near a clinic (5Kilometres radius) and come straight to the hospital without referral letter from the clinic are charged a user fee. If proven that hospital care is better; recommendations will be formulated for policy makers and health care providers to either allow all pregnant mothers with previous caesarean delivery to attend ANC and deliver at the hospital (with a possibility of maternity waiting homes provision), or strengthen the referral system to emergency obstetric and neonatal care facilities, or even empower clinics with comprehensive emergency obstetric and neonatal care capabilities.

## STUDY LIMITATIONS AND POTENTIAL BIAS

The sample and sample size is representative of the population being studied; however, some limitations of this research are listed below.

a) Information bias: hospital records may contain reliable but not always accurate information. The possibility of observer bias can be reduced by developing a standardized data collection tool (with written instructions that allow for the collection of the most appropriate level of detail to be captured). The data will be cross-checked with information kept in relevant registers of deliveries in labour ward and operating theatre. To sensibly minimize potential biases, verification of the information at the primary source (clinics for women referred to NCH) will also be done.

b) Possible confounders such as age, socio-economic status, marital status, and level of education can be controlled by multivariate analysis.

c) This study is limited to those who delivered at the hospital in the group of those who attended antenatal care at the clinic (not including those who attended antenatal care and delivered at the clinic): selection bias. Multivariable logistic regression analysis will be applied.

d) It is also difficult to trace the information on focused (goal directed) antenatal care for these women (both groups) since the details are contained in antenatal cards which are kept by women themselves. A prospective study would answer this challenge. Focused ANC has fewer visits (quality rather than number), but each visit is focused (goal directed) on: detection and management of existing conditions and complications; prevention of complications and diseases; birth preparedness and complications readiness; health promotion.

The reason for previous caesarean is beyond the scope of this study

# References:

1. World health organization: Maternal mortality fact sheet No 348, May 2012. [Online] Available at: http://www.who.int/mediacentre/factsheets/fs348/en/ [accessed 12 March 2014].

2. UNICEF Zambia. Resources-maternal, newborn, and child health. [Online] Available at: http://www.unicef.org/zambia/5109-8457.html [accessed 07 October 2013].

3. UNICEF Zambia. Health, nutrition & HIV and AIDS. [Online] Available at: http://www.org/zambia/health-nutrition.html [accessed 07 October 2013].

4. UNICEF, The state of the world's children 2008. [online] Available at: State of the World's Children, 2008IMR and U5MR for 2008 SOWC [accessed 08 October 2013].

5. World health organization: The final-child-health-situation-summary-Zambia (1). [Online]. Available at: http://www.who.int/entity/bulletin/volumes/86/1/07-043117/eng/-55k [accessed 04 October 2013].

6. Zambia Demographic Health Survey, 2007. [Online] Available at: http://www.nac.org.zm/36-2007-demographic-and-health-survey-zambi... [accessed 06 October 2013].

7. JOÃO PS, CECATTI JG, FAUNDES A et al. Maternal near miss and maternal death in the World Health Organization's 2005 global survey on maternal and perinatal health. [Online] Available at: http://www.who.int/bulletin/volumes/88/2/08-057828.pdf [accessed 04 October 2013].

8. Zambian Ministry of Health. The 2012 list of health facilities in Zambia, Preliminary report, version no. 15. April 2013. [Online] Available at: http://www.moh.gov.zm/index.php/speeches/doc-details/36-the-2012-list-of-health-facilities-in-zambia-preliminary-report.pdf [accessed 09 October 2013].

9. CHANKOVA, SLAVEA and SARA SULZBACH. Zambia Health Services and Systems Program. Occasional Paper Series. Human Resources for Health, Number 1. Bethesda, MD: Health Services and Systems Program, Abt Associates Inc. April 2006. [Online] Available at: http://www.abtassociates.com/reports/HSSP_HRSynthesis1.pdf [accessed 03 October 2013].

10. MOHER D, LIBERATI A, TETZLAFF J, ALTMAN DG. The PRISMA Group (2009). Preferred Reporting Items for Systematic Reviews and Meta-Analyses: The PRISMA Statement. PLoS Med 6(6): e1000097. doi:10.1371/journal.pmed1000097 [Online] Available at: http://www.prisma-statement.org [accessed 29 October 2013].

11. MARK B LANDON. Predicting uterine rupture in women undergoing trial of labour. [Online] Available at: http://www.sciencedirect.com.ezproxy.mmu.ac.uk [accessed 02 November 2013].

12. YUSTER EA. Rethinking the role of the risk approach and antenatal care in maternal mortality reduction. [Online] Available at: http://www.sciencedirect.com.ezproxy.mmu.ac.uk [accessed 02 November 2013].

13. KIM YM, TAPPIS H, ZAINULLAH P et al. Quality of caesarean delivery services and documentation in first line referral facilities in Afghanistan: a chart review. [Online] Available at: http://www.ncbi.nlm.nih.gov/Pubmed... [accessed 03 November 2013].

14. ROSE NM MPEMBENI, KILLEWA JZ, LESHABARI MT et al. Use pattern of maternal health services and determinants of skilled care during delivery in southern Tanzania: implications for achievement of MDG-5 targets. [Online] Available at: http://www.sciencedirect.com.ezproxy.mmu.ac.uk [accessed 02 November 2013].

15. DARMSTAT GL, LEE AC, COUSENS S et al. 60 million non facility births: who can deliver in community settings to reduce intra-partum related deaths? [Online] Available at: http://www.sciencedirect.com.ezproxy.mmu.ac.uk [accessed 02 November 2013].

16. LEE AC, LAWN JE, COUSENS S et al. Linking families and facilities for care at birth: what works to avert intra-partum related deaths? [Online] Available at: http://www.sciencedirect.com.ezproxy.mmu.ac.uk [accessed 02 November 2013].

17. GOUMALATSOS G and VERMA R. Vaginal birth after caesarean section: a practical evidence based approach. [Online] Available at: http://www.sciencedirect.com.ezproxy.mmu.ac.uk [accessed 02 November 2013].

18. RAVI M PATEL and LUCKY J. Delivery after previous caesarean: short term perinatal outcomes. [Online] Available at: http://www.sciencedirect.com.ezproxy.mmu.ac.uk [accessed 02 November 2013].

19. CHIGBU CO, ENNEREJI JO and IKEME AC. Women's experiences following failed vaginal birth after caesarean delivery. [Online] Available at: http://www.sciencedirect.com.ezproxy.mmu.ac.uk [accessed 02 November 2013].

20. MALEDE B and YIRGU G. Factors associated with success of vaginal birth after one caesarean section at three teaching hospitals in Addis Ababa, Ethiopia. [Online] Available at: http://www.ncbi.nlm.nih.gov/Pubmed... [accessed 03 November 2013].

21. WILBERT A SPAANS, VAN DER VELDE FH and ROOSMALEN JV. Trial of labour after previous caesarean section in rural Zimbabwe. . [Online] Available at: http://www.sciencedirect.com.ezproxy.mmu.ac.uk [accessed 02 November 2013].

22. WANYONYI SZ and ROBINSON NK. The utility of clinical pathways in determining perinatal outcomes for women with previous caesarean section. [Online] Available at: http://www.ncbi.nlm.nih.gov/Pubmed... [accessed 03 November 2013].

23. HOFMEYR GJ, HAWS RA, BERGSTROM et al. Obstetric care in low resource settings: what, who, and how to overcome challenges to scale up? [Online] Available at: http://www.sciencedirect.com.ezproxy.mmu.ac.uk [accessed 02 November 2013].

24. ARCHANA S, FAWOLE B, JEMES MM et al. Caesarean delivery outcomes from the WHO global survey on maternal and perinatal health in Africa. [Online] Available at: http://www.sciencedirect.com.ezproxy.mmu.ac.uk [accessed 02 November 2013].

25.CLOKE B and DHARMINTRA PP. Understanding perinatal mortality. [Online] Available at: http://www.sciencedirect.com.ezproxy.mmu.ac.uk [accessed 02 November 2013].

26.FAWOLE AO, SHAH A, TONGO O et al. Determinants of perinatal mortality in Nigeria. [Online] Available at: http://www.sciencedirect.com.ezproxy.mmu.ac.uk [accessed 02 November 2013].

27.ACHARIA S. How effective is antenatal care to promote maternal and neonatal health. [Online] Available at: http://www.sciencedirect.com.ezproxy.mmu.ac.uk [accessed 02 November 2013].

28. BROWN AB, SOHANI SB, KHAN K et al. Antenatal care and perinatal outcomes in Kwale district, Kenya. [Online] Available at: http://www.biomedcentral.com/1471-2393/812 [accessed 04 November 2013].

29. PERVIN J, MORAN A, RAHMAN M et al. Association of antenatal care with facility delivery and perinatal survival: a population based study in Bangladesh. [Online] Available at: http://www.biomedcentral.com/1471-2393/12/111 [accessed 04 November 2013].

30.KAUR J and KAUR K. Does antenatal make a difference? [Online] Available at: http://www.humanbiologyjournal.com/uploads/volume2-Number2-Article2.pdf [accessed 04 November 2013].

31.PRUAL A, TOURE A, HUQUET D et al. The quality of risk factor screening during antenatal consultations in Niger. [Online] Available at: http://www.ncbi.nlm.nih.gov/Pubmed... [accessed 03 November 2013].

32. STEKELENBURG J, KYANAMINA S, MUKELEBAI M et al. Waiting too long: low use of maternal health services in Kalabo, Zambia. [Online] Available at: http://www.sciencedirect.com.ezproxy.mmu.ac.uk [accessed 02 November 2013].

33. BANDA I. Factors associated with late antenatal care attendance in selected rural and urban communities of Copperbelt province, Zambia. [Online] Available at: http://www.hdl.handle.net/123456789/unza.zm [accessed 04 November 2013].

34. KUMBANI LC, CHIRWA E, MALATA A et al. Do Malawian women critically assess the quality of care? A qualitative study on women's perceptions of perinatal care at the district hospital in Malawi. [Online] Available at: http://www.reproductive-health-journal.com/content/9/1/30 [accessed 04 November 2013].

35. ZHAO Q, Huang ZJ, Yang S et al. The utilization of antenatal care among rural to urban migrant women in Shanghai: a hospital based cross sectional study. [Online] Available at: http://www.biomedcentral.com/1471-2458/12/1012 [accessed 04 November 2013].

36. RAHMANI Z and BREKKE M. Antenatal care and obstetric care in Afghanistan: a qualitative study among health care providers. [Online] Available at: http://www.biomedcentral.com/1472-6963/13/166 [accessed 04 November 2013].

37. MAJOKO F. Assessing antenatal care in rural Zimbabwe. [Online] Available at: http://www.diva-portal.org/smash/get/diva2:1671501FULLTEXT01.pdf [accessed 04 November 2013].

38. TULADHAR H and DHAKAL N. Impact of antenatal care on maternal and perinatal outcome: a study at Nepal medical college teaching hospital. [Online] Available at: http://www.nepjol.info/index.php/NJOG/article/view6755 [accessed 04 November 2013].

39. BANDA C. Barriers to utilization of focused antenatal care among pregnant women in Ntchisi district in Malawi. [Online] Available at: http://www.tampub.uta.fi/bitstream/handle/10024/84640/... [accessed 04 November 2013].

40. CARROLI G, ROONEY C, and VILLAR J. How effective is antenatal care in preventing maternal mortality and serious morbidity? An overview of the evidence. [Online] Available at: http://www.sciencedirect.com.ezproxy.mmu.ac.uk [accessed 02 November 2013].

41. NICHOLAS NA KYEI. Quality of antenatal care in Zambia: a national assessment. [Online] Available at: http://www.biomedcentral.com/1471-2393/12/151/... [accessed 04 November 2013].

42. World Health Organization. Ndola, Zambia – London, England. [Online] Available at: http://www. who.int/patientsafety/implementation/apps/first_wave/ndola_london/en/ - 25k [accessed 10 April 2014].

43. Zambia/World bank –Trading Economics. Birth rate – crude (per 1; 000 people) in Zambia. [Online] Available at: http://www.tradingeconomics.com/Zambia/birth-rate-crude-per-1-000-people-... [accessed 10 April 2014].

44. FLEIS JL. Statistical methods for rates and proportions. New York: John Wiley and sons, 1981.pp44-45 [Online] Available at: http://www. slideshare.net/drtamil/6-calculate-samplesize-for-cohort-studies [accessed 10 April 2014].

# APPENDIX I SUMMARY OF THE ARTICLES IDENTIFIED FOR REVIEW

| No | AUTHOR | TITLE | COUNTRY | YEAR | TYPE OF STUDY | SAMPLING METHOD | MAIN RESULTS/RELEVANCE | CRITICAL COMMENT |
|---|---|---|---|---|---|---|---|---|
| 1 | Darmstadt GL. et al.[15] | 60 million non facility births: who can deliver in community settings to reduce intra-partum related deaths? | – | 2009 | Systematic review | Secondary data analysis | . Low quality evidence for skilled birth attendance provision in the community. | High grade study in the hierarchy of evidence. The study does not look at skilled birth attendants only, but also at other community cadres such as traditional birth attendants and community health workers. |
| 2 | Anne CC Lee et al.[16] | Linking families and facilities for care at birth: what works to avert intra-partum related deaths? | – | 2009 | Systematic review | Secondary data analysis | . Moderate quality evidence: community awareness and participation can increase delivery at health facilities and decrease significantly perinatal mortalities. | High grade study in the hierarchy of evidence. The impact of promising but limited evidence (on financial schemes and referral systems in the community) on mortality is not known. |
| 3 | Franz Majoko[37] | Assessing antenatal care in rural Zimbabwe | Zimbabwe | 2005 | Cluster randomized controlled trial | A cluster randomized controlled trial was carried out in Gutu rural (Zimbabwe) to evaluate a 5 goal oriented antenatal care against the standard model of care | . The new model did not influence antenatal visits, rather improved the use of health care . The classical risk screening model had low predictive value and large risk group for referral . Multiparous mothers with previous complications had increased chances of complications but | Randomization was possible using health centre as a unit of randomization though an individualised controlled trial could have been preferred. The study can still suffer selection and observer bias. |

| | | | | | | | improved health care services and reduced negative perinatal outcomes | |
|---|---|---|---|---|---|---|---|---|
| 4 | Prual A et al.[31] | The quality of risk factor screening during antenatal consultations in Niger | Niger | 2000 | Qualitative cohort study | Random selection of 330 pregnant mothers attending antenatal consultations in 8 maternal and child health centres in two urban areas and one rural town in Niger | . Poor quality risk factors screening .55% of pregnant women had 1 risk factor or more .31% had more than one risk factors . 99% of risk factors were detected at interview. Midwives did not systematically search for risk factors/height, BP, glycosuria, vaginal bleeding, oedema, parity, age, previous caesarean, previous stillbirths or miscarriages | Good quality evidence study. The sample randomization helped to control possible confounders. The sample representation increases also the external validity (in relation to the Zambian populations) of this study. |
| 5 | Celia AB. Et al.[28] | Antenatal care and perinatal outcomes in Kwale district, Kenya | Kenya | 2008 | A cohort survey | A cohort survey of 1.562 perinatal outcomes(2004-2005) in the catchment areas for 5 ministry of health dispensaries in two divisions of the Kwale region | . 32% of women reported having any ANC . The number of ANC visits increase with distance from the dispensary(paradoxically): OR 1.46; 95%CI 1.33-1.60 . Women attending ANC at least twice were more likely to have a live birth and were more likely to have a healthy weigh baby | The quality of data: it can be difficult to obtain accurate estimates of catchment areas or target populations through this method(continuous or routine data collection) |

Table 3: summary of reviewed articles

| No | AUTHOR | TITLE | COUNTRY | YEAR | TYPE OF STUDY | SAMPLING METHOD | MAIN RESULTS/RELEVANCE | CRITICAL COMMENT |
|---|---|---|---|---|---|---|---|---|
| 6 | Tuladhar H. And Dhakal N.[38] | Impact of antenatal care on maternal and perinatal outcome: a | Nepal | 2011 | Prospective descriptive study | 322 women who had delivered at Nepal medical | . 87% of women had adequate antenatal care . 6.5% of women did not attend antenatal | Well described pattern, quality and determinants of antenatal care attendance in the |

| | | | | | | | | |
|---|---|---|---|---|---|---|---|---|
| | | study at Nepal medical college teaching hospital | | | | college teaching hospital- were included in the prospective study (April to August 2010). | care . Most women preferred to attend antenatal care at the hospital . Caesarean section rate: 17.4% mostly in those who received antenatal care . Maternal and perinatal complications were common in the group of women with inadequate antennal care. | studied population. |
| 7 | Malede B and Yirgu G.[20] | Factors associated with success of vaginal birth after one caesarean section at three teaching hospitals in Addis Ababa, Ethiopia | Ethiopia | 2013 | Case control study | Comparison of VBAC risk factors in 3 teaching hospitals. Cases: 101 successful vaginal deliveries. Controls: 103 unsuccessful VBAC and delivered by caesarean section. Between May 2009 and May 2010 | . History of past successful VBAC, ruptured membranes and dilated cervix (more than 3Cm) at admission were determinants for successful VBAC . Labour dysfunction was the commonest reason for repeat caesarean after trial of labour | Moderate grade of evidence. Good study design (at the specialist level of care) with good choice of cases and controls. |
| 8 | Wilbert AS, Van der Velde FH and Roosmalen JV.[21] | Trial of labour after previous caesarean section in rural Zimbabwe | Zimbabwe | 1996 | Case control study | All pregnant women with a previous caesarean (delivered between January 1991 and December | . 44% of mothers delivered vaginally after caesarean . One uterine scar rupture secondary to thyrotoxicosis . No significant perinatal and maternal results | There is a possibility of observation bias. Also ethical issues: not offering an option of elective caesarean section in women with previous caesarean delivery plus co-morbidities such as |

| | | | | | | | | |
|---|---|---|---|---|---|---|---|---|
| | | | | | | 1993) at Mnene District hospital. Outcome of 281 women with one or more caesarean was compared with 4501 women who had not previously delivered by caesarean | difference in the two groups . The risk of repeat caesarean was significantly increased for CPD . Planned caesarean after caesarean delivery: none | thyrotoxicosis (resulting in uterine rupture). |
| 9 | Adeniran OF, Archana S. et al.[26] | Determinants of perinatal mortality in Nigeria | Nigeria | 2011 | Cross sectional study | Stratified multistage cluster sampling of 21 health settings registering more than 1000 births per year selected. Information collected on all mothers who delivered and their new born infants( within a period of three months) | . Mother' age, lack of antenatal care, un-booked status, prematurity and asphyxia at birth are predictors of perinatal deaths. . Stillbirth rate: 71 per 1000 deliveries, Perinatal mortality rate: 78 per 1000 deliveries, early neonatal mortality rate: 8 per 1000 deliveries, birth weight less than 2500g: 10%, birth before 37 weeks of gestation:12.3% | . Strong study design: prospective data collection and follow up of delivered women and their infants in nationally representative health facilities |
| 10 | Kim YM, Tappis H, Zainullah P et al.[13] | Quality of caesarean delivery services and documentation | Afghanistan | 2012 | Cross sectional study | Descriptive evaluation of 173 caesarean section | . No caesarean performed in the previous 3 months at lower level health settings | . Moderate grade of evidence . Possible risk of information(contained in hospital records) |

| | | | | | | | | bias |
|---|---|---|---|---|---|---|---|---|
| | in first line referral facilities in Afghanistan: a chart review | | | | deliveries in 62 first line emergency obstetric and neonatal care(EmONC) facilities serving as referral( based on review of record) | . Most caesarean section deliveries(88%) were emergencies . 12% were referred from another facility . Among 173 documented cases: 27 maternal mortalities, 28 stillbirths, and 3 early neonatal mortalities | | |

Table 3 (continued)

| No | AUTHOR | TITLE | COUNTRY | YEAR | TYPE OF STUDY | SAMPLING METHOD | MAIN RESULTS/RELEVANCE | CRITICAL COMMENT |
|---|---|---|---|---|---|---|---|---|
| 11 | Isaac Banda[33] | Factors associated with late antenatal care attendance in selected rural and urban communities of the Copperbelt province, Zambia | Zambia | 2012 | Cross sectional study | A semi-structured questionnaire was conducted in selected health facilities of Mpongwe rural district(307 women attending antenatal clinic) and Ndola urban district(306 women attending antenatal clinic) | . Prevalence of ANC attendance 72.0%. the difference between the two districts was not statistically significant . Women in urban district had adequate knowledge about ANC. This is 2.2 times high odds for early attendance of ANC than women who had inadequate knowledge | There is possibility of information bias. Recall bias in not nullified when administering such questionnaire. Especially in rural Zambia where education level is low. |
| 12 | Lily C. Kumbani et al.[34] | Do Malawian women critically assess the quality of care? A qualitative study on | Malawi | 2012 | Cross sectional descriptive study | Data were collected qualitatively by in depth interviews (14) using face to face semi-structured | . Mothers desired to be treated well (received with respect, kindness, dignity, privacy, confidentiality and not shouted at). . Mothers were not critical at the received | Small sample size that might not be representative of the population being studied (hospital based and not population based |

| | | women's perceptions of perinatal care at a district hospital in Malawi | | | | questionnaires to mothers who delivered normally at Chiradzulu district hospital (February 2011- March 2011) | care (lack of awareness on standard of care). | survey). The study might also suffer information bias (interviews conducted within the hospital). Altogether, qualitative study. |
|---|---|---|---|---|---|---|---|---|
| 13 | Jesmin Pervin et al.[29] | Association of antenatal care with facility delivery and perinatal survival-a population based study in Bangladesh | Bangladesh | 2012 | Population based survey | Data were prospectively collected using ongoing health and demographic surveillance system, and the newly completed maternal, neonatal and child health program. Pregnant women were identified at their homes and followed up routinely. | Antenatal care attendance was associated with increased delivery at health facilities and substantial reduction in perinatal mortality. | Strengths: being a population based survey; data were collected prospectively in two areas. Weaknesses: non randomization, the comparison between the two areas being difficult. |
| 14 | Qi Zhao et al.[35] | The utilization of antenatal care among rural to urban migrant women in Shanghai: a hospital based cross sectional study | China | 2012 | Cross sectional study – hospital based | Women who migrated to Shanghai, lived there for more than 6 months and delivered at the hospital (August2009 – February 2010) were selected. A structured questionnaire was used for interviews. | . 90.1% of women had at least one antenatal visit . 49.7% of women had adequate (5 or more visits) antenatal care . Older women had adequate antenatal care compared with the younger ones (below 25 years). 19.7% of women had antenatal care during first trimester. | The generalisability- external validity of the findings of this study is limited (hospital based survey of a specific group of population). The study design does not allow establishing the causes of underutilization of antenatal care in this population. |

| 15 | Japinder Kaur and Kawaljit Kaur[30] | Does antenatal make a difference? | India | 2013 | Retrospective survey | Women who had ANC and delivered at Punjab (institute of medical science) were included. Structured questionnaires were used to interview participants after delivery. Data were compared with that of those who delivered at the same institution but did not attend ANC there (April-June 2012). | . 42% of women were booked for antenatal care .58% of women were referred from other health facilities. The required antenatal care was missing in this group. There were also increased obstetric complications among them. | The definition of un-booked mothers is not clear: including those without antenatal care during their whole pregnancy and those referred from other health facilities (emergencies). It is not clear whether these emergencies had antenatal care at their referring institutions or not. |

Table 3 (continued)

| No | AUTHOR | TITLE | COUNTRY | YEAR | TYPE OF STUDY | SAMPLING METHOD | MAIN RESULTS/RELEVANCE | CRITICAL COMMENT |
|---|---|---|---|---|---|---|---|---|
| 16 | Chigbu CO, Ennereji JO and Ikeme AC.[19] | Women's experiences following failed vaginal birth after caesarean delivery | Nigeria | 2007 | Cross sectional study | Prested questions ( both open and closed ended) self administered - to participants awaiting antenatal check up (January 2002 to June 2006) | . Women who had successful vaginal delivery reported a positive experience. Those who failed to deliver vaginally had a negative experience. They reported limitations in available options-making it uneasy to attempt vaginal delivery after caesarean. | The sample may not be representative of the population studied. The study may also be biased by a possibility of recall/information bias |
| 17 | Rose NM Mpembeni | Use pattern of maternal | Tanzania | 2007 | Cross sectional | A random sample of 974 | . Almost all women (99.8%) had attended | Good control of confounders by |

| | | | | | | | | |
|---|---|---|---|---|---|---|---|---|
| | et al.[14] | health services and determinants of skilled care during delivery in southern Tanzania: implications for achievement of MDG-5 targets | | | study | women (aged 14 to 50 years) who delivered within one year before the survey. They were interviewed ( structured questionnaire) in Mtwara rural district | 1 or more ANC (during last pregnancy). . 46.7% of them only delivered at health institution. . 44.5% only had skilled birth assistance. . Factors associated with significant use of skilled birth assistance: distance, male partner involvement (discussion on place of delivery and obstetric risks). | randomization (a multistage cluster random sampling method was used). The sample is also relevant to the Zambian population. |
| 18 | Stekelenburg J. Et al.[32] | Waiting too long: low use of maternal health services in Kalabo, Zambia | Zambia | 2004 | Cross sectional descriptive study | 332 women were interviewed using semi-structured questionnaires in Kalabo district between 1998 and 2000 | . 96% of participants preferred clinic delivery . 54% of participants delivered at the clinic. Reasons: distance, staff insufficiency and deficiency, lack of equipment at health facilities | Very relevant study for the research. The researcher combines both quantitative and qualitative methods-complementing each other. |
| 19 | Archana S, Fawole B, Jemes MM. Et al.[24] | Caesarean delivery outcomes from the WHO global survey on maternal and perinatal health in Africa | Algeria, Angola, Congo, Kenya, Niger, Nigeria and Uganda | 2009 | Cross sectional study | Data obtained from all women delivered (83439 births) in chosen health settings (131) in Africa (7 countries): September 2004 - March 2005. By trained staff - within 24 hours | . Median caesarean delivery rate: 8.8% . Caesarean deliveries performed only in 95 facilities (73%) . Adjusted emergency caesarean raised the risk of maternal and neonatal deaths, fresh stillbirths and extreme sickness of the neonate . Adjusted elective caesarean delivery rate: fewer perinatal mortalities . Emergency caesarean: often too late to avert perinatal | Strong evidence and generalisability to the Zambian setting. Increased emergency caesareans were associated with negative perinatal outcomes as compared with planned caesareans. Potential confounders were adjusted. |

| | | | | | | | mortalities | |
|---|---|---|---|---|---|---|---|---|
| 20 | Christina Leah Banda[39] | Barriers to utilization of focused antenatal care among pregnant women in Ntchisi district in Malawi | Malawi | 2013 | Cross sectional quantitative study | Structured questionnaires were administered to pregnant women (120), postnatal women (84) and health workers (36) from 12 facilities in Ntchisi district | . 96% of participants (women) knew something about focused antenatal care . High parity women, long distance, seeking permission, beliefs such as witchcraft, and women aged 20 to 25 years: were associated with low utilization of focused antenatal care . Health workers perceived focused antenatal care positively. | The study was based at the health facilities and not at the population level. There is also risk of recall bias among participating women. Confounders are not controlled (when analysing the findings of the study). |

Table 3 (continued)

| No | AUTHOR | TITLE | COUNTRY | YEAR | TYPE OF STUDY | SAMPLING METHOD | MAIN RESULTS/RELEVANCE | CRITICAL COMMENT |
|---|---|---|---|---|---|---|---|---|
| 21 | Zuhal Rahmani and Mette Brekke[36] | Antenatal and obstetric care in Afghanistan – a qualitative study among health care providers | Afghanistan | 2013 | Cross sectional qualitative study | Semi-structured questionnaires were used to interview 27 people (12 pregnant and postnatal women, 7 doctors, 5 midwives and 3 traditional birth attendants) in two provinces of Afghanistan (2010) at health facilities or participant homes. | There was underuse of antenatal care services even though available. Lack of knowledge, financial challenges, health workers' attitudes, and poor working conditions were among identified obstacles to antenatal care services. | . Qualitative study. . Small sample size that might not be representative of the population being studied – limiting the external validity of the study . Questionnaire was administered in the local language. Language barrier could have influenced the translation of the information. |

| 22 | Ravi M Patel and Lucky J.[18] | Delivery after previous caesarean: Short-Term perinatal outcomes | US | 2010 | Seminars in Perinatology | Secondary data analysis | . RCT comparing vaginal birth after caesarean and elective repeat caesarean are lacking . Observational studies suggest an increased risk of perinatal death and hypoxic ischemic encephalopathy(in trial of labour): rare risks . Less severe increased respiratory morbidity (in elective caesarean): common risks | Low grade study in the hierarchy of evidence but very relevant to this research. |
|---|---|---|---|---|---|---|---|---|
| 23 | Mark B Landon[11] | Predicting uterine rupture in women undergoing trial of labour | – | 2010 | Seminars in perinatology | Secondary data analysis | . Absolute risk of uterine rupture in trial of labour after caesarean delivery: 0.5 to 4% . Low risk factors: previous vaginal delivery, prior successful vaginal birth after caesarean . High risk factors: multiple prior caesareans, short inter-pregnancy interval, single layer uterine closure, prior preterm caesarean, labour induction and augmentation | Low grade study in the hierarchy of evidence but very relevant to this research as demonstrated beside. |
| 24 | Wanyonyi SZ and Robinson NK.[22] | The utility of clinical pathways in determining perinatal outcomes for women with one previous caesarean section | Kenya | 2010 | Review of records( retrospective study) | Retrospective evaluation of case delivery notes and records. At the Agakhan University hospital ( between January 2008 and December 2009) | . A total 215 previous caesarean mothers assessed following the standard pathway for care . 46 percent of them, being eligible, chose a trial of labour. 49.9 percent had a successful vaginal birth after caesarean. .Conforming maternal | The sample might not be representative of the population being studied. Hospital records may contain valid but not always accurate information. |

| No | AUTHOR | TITLE | COUNTRY | YEAR | TYPE OF STUDY | SAMPLING METHOD | MAIN RESULTS/RELEVANCE | CRITICAL COMMENT |
|---|---|---|---|---|---|---|---|---|
| | | | | | | | morbidity results for successful and failed vaginal delivery after caesarean. | |
| 25 | Yuster EA.[12] | Rethinking the role of the risk approach and ANC in maternal mortality reduction | India | 1995 | Case scenario | Hypothetical example of 7750 pregnant women with maternal mortality ratio of 12.9 per 1000 live births(250 high risk women) | . ANC can contribute to preventing maternal deaths: detecting danger and educating mothers on obstetric complications. Motivate mothers and their families to inquire for referral care when appropriate.<br>. Obstetric risk approach is neither cost effective nor efficient in developing settings | Low grade in the hierarchy of evidence but relevant to the study. |

Table 3 (continued)

| No | AUTHOR | TITLE | COUNTRY | YEAR | TYPE OF STUDY | SAMPLING METHOD | MAIN RESULTS/RELEVANCE | CRITICAL COMMENT |
|---|---|---|---|---|---|---|---|---|
| 26 | Cloke B. and Dharmintra P P.[25] | Understanding perinatal mortality. | _ | 2013 | Literature review | Secondary data analysis | . Uterine rupture associated with vaginal delivery after caesarean birth, modest obstetric units and place of birth are determinants of risk factors for term delivery related perinatal deaths. | . Limited statistical information<br>. Relative risk estimation(for individual risk factors) not established |
| 27 | Goumalatsos G. And Varma R.[17] | Vaginal birth after caesarean section: a practical evidence based approach | _ | 2009 | Literature review | Secondary data analysis | . Individualised complete informed consent on risk/benefits on planned vaginal birth after caesarean( VBAC) or elective repeat caesarean section(ERCS) for women with previous caesarean delivery is important<br>. Planned VBAC is associated with high | High evidence and practical approach to antenatal care and intra-partum care for women with previous caesarean section |

| | | | | | | | maternal and perinatal morbidity/mortality | |
|---|---|---|---|---|---|---|---|---|
| 28 | Justus GH. Et al.[23] | Obstetric care in low resource settings: what, who, and how to overcome challenges to scale up? | – | 2009 | Literature review | Secondary data analysis | . Limited evidence on intra-partum interventions to reduce intra-partum related neonatal mortality or morbidity . Planned caesarean for breech presentation and post term induction may be unavailable or less safe in low resource settings and require risk benefit assessment | There is possibility of information bias. Most of the reviewed evidence was very low or low grade in the hierarchy of evidence, with little moderate grade evidence. |
| 29 | Guillermo C. et al.[40] | How effective is antenatal care in preventing maternal mortality and serious morbidity? An overview of the evidence | – | 2001 | Literature review | Secondary data analysis | An overview of evidence of the effectiveness of ANC in relation to maternal mortality and serious morbidity (in developing settings): Little is known. | Quality evidence study with a particular focus on developing settings (including critical review of scientific evidence of randomised controlled trials and observational studies). |
| 30 | Acharya S.[27] | How effective is antenatal care to promote maternal and neonatal health | – | 1995 | Literature review | Secondary data analysis | . ANC is effective, but relies strongly on the attitude of health personnel . Community participation and family members involvement is necessary for ANC promotion . Transport to well equipped facilities for emergency obstetric care is essential | Provides strong evidence of relevance to the research. Reviewing major causes of maternal mortality and morbidity, and how antenatal care can effectively help reduce them. |

Table 3 (continued)

| No | AUTHOR | TITLE | COUNTRY | YEAR | TYPE OF STUDY | SAMPLING METHOD | MAIN RESULTS/RELEVANCE | CRITICAL COMMENT |
|---|---|---|---|---|---|---|---|---|
| 31 | Nicholas NA Kyei[41] | Quality of antenatal care in Zambia: a national assessment | Zambia | 2012 | Literature review | Secondary data analysis | . 3% of ANC fulfilled the developed criteria for optimum ANC service . 47% provided adequate service . 50% offered inadequate service . Only 29% of mothers received good quality ANC, and only 8% of mothers received good quality ANC and attended in the first trimester | The study demonstrates clearly the gap in existing Zambian national data on antenatal care coverage-needing focused quality antenatal care. However, there is possibility of measurement bias. |
| | | | | | | | | |
| | | | | | | | | |
| | | | | | | | | |
| | | | | | | | | |

Table 3 (continued)

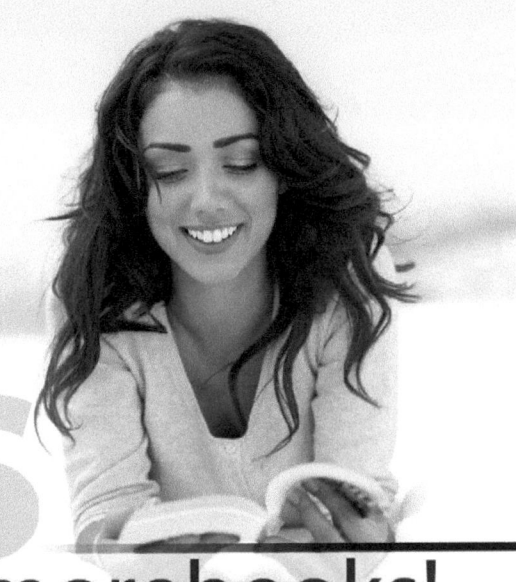
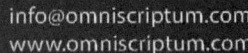
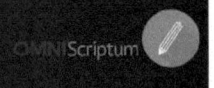

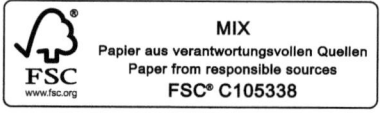
Printed by Books on Demand GmbH, Norderstedt / Germany